Spinal Stenosis Diet

A Beginner's Quick Start Guide to Managing the Condition Through Diet and Other Lifestyle Remedies, With Sample Recipes

PATRICK MARSHWELL

Disclaimer

By reading this disclaimer, you are accepting the terms of the disclaimer in full. If you disagree with this disclaimer, please do not read the guide.

All of the content within this guide is provided for informational and educational purposes only, and should not be accepted as independent medical or other professional advice. The author is not a doctor, physician, nurse, mental health provider, or registered nutritionist/dietician. Therefore, using and reading this guide does not establish any form of a physician-patient relationship.

Always consult with a physician or another qualified health provider with any issues or questions you might have regarding any sort of medical condition. Do not ever disregard any qualified professional medical advice or delay seeking that advice because of anything you have read in this guide. The information in this guide is not intended to be any sort of medical advice and should not be used in lieu of any medical advice by a licensed and qualified medical professional.

The information in this guide has been compiled from a variety of known sources. However, the author cannot attest to or guarantee the accuracy of each source and thus should not be held liable for any errors or omissions.

Introduction

Spinal stenosis is a condition in which the spaces in the spine narrow, placing pressure on the spinal cord and nerves. This can lead to pain, numbness, and weakness in the arms or legs. Spinal stenosis is most often caused by age-related changes in the spine, such as the development of arthritis.

However, it can also be caused by other conditions, such as tumors or injuries. In some cases, spinal stenosis may be present at birth. Treatment for spinal stenosis typically involves medications to relieve pain and other symptoms.

In severe cases, surgery may be necessary to widen the spaces in the spine and relieve pressure on the nerves.

In this quick guide we will discuss the following in detail:

- What are the 2 types of spinal stenosis?
- What causes spinal stenosis?
- What are the symptoms of spinal stenosis?
- When to see a doctor?
- How is spinal stenosis diagnosed?
- What are the medical treatments for spinal stenosis?
- How to prevent spinal stenosis?
- How to manage symptoms of spinal stenosis using natural methods?

- How to manage symptoms of spinal stenosis through diet?

So, let's get started.

Table of Contents

THE TWO TYPES OF SPINAL STENOSIS

Spinal stenosis is a condition that occurs when the spinal canal narrows, placing pressure on the spinal cord and nerves. There are two main types of spinal stenosis: cervical and lumbar.

Cervical spinal stenosis: Cervical spinal stenosis is a degenerative condition that affects the spinal cord and nerves in the neck. The condition is caused by the narrowing of the spinal canal, which puts pressure on the spinal cord and nerves. This can lead to pain, numbness, and weakness in the arms and legs. In severe cases, it can also lead to paralysis.

Lumbar spinal stenosis: Lumbar spinal stenosis occurs when the spinal canal narrows in the lower back. This narrowing can put pressure on the spinal cord and nerves, causing pain, numbness, and weakness in the legs. In severe cases, it can lead to paralysis. Lumbar spinal stenosis is most common in people over the age of 50. It is more likely to occur in people who have had a previous spine injury or who have a family history of the condition.

What Causes Spinal Stenosis?

Spinal stenosis is a condition that manifests when the spinal canal narrows and puts pressure on the spinal cord and nerve roots. This can happen due to several reasons.

Age-related changes in the spine: Spinal stenosis is caused by age-related changes in the spine. These changes can include the thinning of the bones and the deterioration of the disks between the vertebrae. The disks act as cushions, and as they deteriorate, they lose their ability to absorb shocks. This can lead to pain and other symptoms.

Tumors: Tumors are one possible cause of spinal stenosis. Tumors can form anywhere in the body, including the spine. While most tumors are benign, or noncancerous, some may be cancerous. Whether benign or cancerous, tumors can cause the spine to narrow, leading to spinal stenosis.

In some cases, tumors may be removed surgically. If the tumor is cancerous, additional treatment, such as radiation or chemotherapy, may be necessary. If you have been diagnosed with a tumor in your spine, work with your doctor to develop a treatment plan that is right for you.

Injuries: When the spine is injured, it may heal in a way that narrows the spinal canal. This can occur due to the formation of scar tissue, the displacement of bones or disks, or other changes in the structure of the spine.

In some cases, spinal stenosis may also be caused by birth defects or degenerative changes that occur with age. While injuries are a common cause of this condition, it is important to remember that not everyone who experiences an injury will go on to develop spinal stenosis.

If you have experienced an injury and are experiencing symptoms such as pain, numbness, or weakness, it is important to seek medical attention so that a proper diagnosis can be made.

Herniated Discs: One of the primary causes of spinal stenosis is herniated discs. A herniated disc occurs when the soft inner material of the disc leaks out through a tear in the outer layer. This can put pressure on the spinal cord or nerves, leading to pain, numbness, and weakness. In some cases, a herniated disc can also cause spinal stenosis by narrowing the spinal canal. Herniated discs are often the result of wear and tear on the discs, which can occur with age.

Birth defects: One of the most common causes of Spinal Stenosis is birth defects. Birth defects can cause the bones in the spine to fuse or grow abnormally. This can lead to a narrowing of the spinal canal, which can put pressure on the nerves.

Scheuermann's disease: Scheuermann's disease is a disorder of the spine that is characterized by the abnormal development of the vertebrae. The result of this is a deformity of the spine that can lead to a narrowing of the spinal canal. In severe cases, this can compress the spinal cord and nerves, causing pain, numbness, and weakness in the legs.

SYMPTOMS OF SPINAL STENOSIS

The symptoms of spinal stenosis vary depending on the type and severity of the condition.

Cervical spinal stenosis can cause:

Pain in the neck, shoulders, and arms: The pain is caused by the compression of the spinal cord or nerves in the neck. The symptoms can vary from mild to severe, and they may come and go. In some cases, the pain may be constant. The pain may be worse when you are active or when you bend your neck.

Numbness or weakness in the arms: In some cases, the symptoms may be mild and only occur when the person is engaged in activities that put pressure on the spine, such as lifting weights. However, in other cases, the symptoms can be much more severe and may even cause paralysis.

Difficulty walking: One of the most common symptoms of cervical spinal stenosis is difficulty walking. This is caused by the narrowing of the spinal canal, which puts pressure on the spinal cord and nerves. The pressure can cause pain, numbness, and weakness in the arms and legs. It can also make it difficult to walk or stand for long periods. In severe cases, cervical spinal stenosis can lead to paralysis.

Loss of balance: Many people with cervical spinal stenosis experience loss of balance. This is because the spinal cord is responsible for sending signals from the brain to the rest of the body. When there is pressure on the spinal cord, these signals can be interrupted, causing problems with movement and balance.

Lumbar spinal stenosis can cause:

Pain in the lower back and legs: Symptoms of lumbar spinal stenosis include pain in the lower back and legs, numbness or weakness in the legs, and difficulty walking. The pain is caused by pressure on the nerves within the spinal canal. In severe cases, lumbar spinal stenosis can lead to paralysis.

Numbness or weakness in the legs: Lumbar spinal stenosis is a condition in which the spinal canal narrows, placing pressure on the nerves that travel through it. This pressure can lead to a variety of symptoms, including numbness or weakness in the legs. In some cases, these symptoms may only occur when walking or standing for long periods. However, as the condition progresses, they may become constant.

Difficulty walking: One of the most common symptoms is difficulty walking. This may occur because the narrowing of the spinal canal puts pressure on the nerves that control leg movement. As a result, patients may find it difficult to lift their legs or walk for long periods.

Loss of balance: One of the less common symptoms of lumbar spinal stenosis is a loss of balance. This can be due to the compression of the nerves in the spine, which can interfere with the signals that are sent to the brain regarding balance. In some cases, this may only happen when the individual is standing for long periods or walking. However, in more severe cases, it may happen even when sitting or lying down. Loss of balance can lead to falls, which can result in serious injuries. Therefore, it is important to be aware of this symptom and to seek medical help if it occurs.

When to See a Doctor?

If you experience any of the above symptoms, it is important to see a doctor for a diagnosis. Spinal stenosis can be difficult to diagnose because the symptoms can mimic other conditions, such as herniated discs or arthritis.

Your doctor will likely order imaging tests, such as an MRI or CT scan, to confirm the diagnosis.

DIAGNOSING AND TREATING SPINAL STENOSIS

Spinal stenosis is diagnosed through a combination of medical history, physical examination, and imaging tests.

Your doctor may order one or more of the following tests to diagnose spinal stenosis:

Physical Examination: Your doctor will likely perform a physical examination to look for signs of spinal stenosis. This may include checking for pain, numbness, or weakness in your back, neck, or legs.

X-ray: An X-ray can often show whether there is a narrowing of the spinal canal or degenerative changes in the spine that may be causing symptoms. If an X-ray does not provide enough information, other imaging tests such as an MRI or CT scan may be recommended.

MRI: The best way to look at the spine is with an MRI. The MRI can show the shape of the spinal canal and whether it is narrowed. An MRI also can show herniated discs and tumors. In some cases, your doctor may order a special type of MRI that uses a contrast dye. The dye makes it easier to see certain structures in your spine.

CT scan: A CT scan is often used to get a detailed look at the spine and identify any areas of narrowing.

Myelogram: In this test, a dye is injected into the spinal canal. This dye helps to better visualize the spinal cord and nerves on an X-ray or CT scan.

Spinal tap: Sometimes doctors use a needle to take out a small amount of fluid from around your spinal cord or nerves (spinal tap). They can then look at the fluid under a microscope for signs of infections, inflammation, or other problems.

What are the medical treatments for spinal stenosis?

Treatment for spinal stenosis depends on the severity of the condition. In mild cases, treatment may only be necessary to relieve symptoms.

Medications: Treatment for spinal stenosis typically focuses on relieving symptoms and preventing the condition from progressing. Medications that may be used to treat this condition include pain relievers, anti-inflammatory drugs, nerve blockers, and steroids.

Physical therapy: Physical therapy is one such treatment. Physical therapists can provide exercises and stretches that help to improve flexibility and relieve pain. They can also teach patients how to properly use assistive devices such as canes or walkers. In addition, physical therapists can develop an individualized exercise program that helps to maintain mobility and prevent further decline.

Epidural injections: Also known as epidural steroid injections, these injections are designed to reduce inflammation and pain in the spine. The medication is injected directly into the epidural space, which is the area around the spinal cord.

Epidural injections are effective in treating a wide range of conditions, including herniated disks, pinched nerves, and degenerative disk disease. In most cases, patients can expect to see an improvement in their symptoms within a few days of receiving an injection.

However, it is important to note that epidural injections are not a cure for spinal stenosis. Rather, they are intended to provide relief from the symptoms of the condition.

Surgery: Surgery is typically recommended for those who have not responded well to other forms of treatment, such as physical therapy or medication. The goal of surgery is to relieve pressure on the spinal cord or nerves by widening the spinal canal or removing excess tissue. While surgery is often successful in relieving pain and restoring mobility, it is also a major procedure that carries a risk of complications. As such, it should only be considered after all other options have been exhausted.

PREVENTION OF SPINAL STENOSIS

There is no sure way to prevent spinal stenosis. However, there are some things you can do to reduce your risk:

Maintain a healthy weight: Maintaining a healthy weight is one of the best things you can do to prevent spinal stenosis. Excess weight puts extra pressure on your spine, which can lead to the formation of bone spurs and other changes that narrow the spaces between the bones in your spine. Losing weight can help to reduce this pressure and prevent spinal stenosis from developing or getting worse.

Exercise regularly: Exercise is one of the best ways to keep your spine healthy. Strengthening the muscles around the spine can help to take pressure off of the vertebrae and prevent the formation of bone spurs. In addition, maintaining good posture and avoiding activities that put unnecessary strain on the spine can also help to prevent this condition. If you are at risk of developing spinal stenosis, talk to your doctor about ways you can reduce your risk.

Stop smoking: The nicotine in cigarettes damages the tissues in your spine, causing them to swell and put pressure on your spinal cord. In addition, smoking decreases blood flow to the spine, which can further damage the tissue. If you smoke and are experiencing back pain, see your doctor. Quitting smoking is the best way to prevent this condition from worsening.

NATURAL METHODS TO MANAGE THE SYMPTOMS OF SPINAL STENOSIS

There are a few things you can do at home to help manage your symptoms:

Apply heat or ice: While there is no definitive cure for this pain, some people find relief by applying heat or ice to the affected area. The heat can help improve blood circulation and loosen up stiff muscles. The ice can help numb the area and reduce inflammation.

It's important to experiment to see what works best for you and to be careful not to overdo it. Applying too much heat or ice can cause skin damage. If you're not sure how to proceed, consult a doctor or physical therapist for guidance.

Acupuncture: Acupuncture is a Traditional Chinese Medicine technique that involves inserting thin needles into the skin at specific points on the body. Some people find that it helps relieve pain caused by conditions like spinal stenosis, fibromyalgia, and migraines.

The exact mechanism by which acupuncture works is still not fully understood, but it is thought to stimulate the nervous system and release endorphins, which are natural pain relievers.

Acupuncture is generally considered to be safe when performed by a trained professional, and side effects are typically mild and temporary. Some people also find that acupuncture helps to improve their overall sense of well-being.

Massage therapy: Massage therapy is an effective treatment for reducing muscle tension and pain caused by spinal stenosis. Massage therapy can help to release the pressure on the spinal cord and nerves, improving mobility and reducing pain. In addition, massage therapy can help to improve circulation and increase the range of motion. As a result, massage therapy can be an important part of treatment for people with spinal stenosis.

Stretch and do a range of motion exercises: When it comes to spinal stenosis, several things can help alleviate the symptoms and improve your quality of life. One of those things is maintaining a good range of motion in your spine. This can be done through a variety of exercises and stretches that help keep your spine flexible.

Additionally, spinal stenosis often leads to a loss of muscle mass in the affected area. This loss of muscle can further limit your range of motion and increase pain levels. As such, it is important to maintain strong muscles around your spine through regular exercise. By doing so, you can help improve your flexibility and reduce the pain associated with spinal stenosis.

Practice good posture: Posture plays an important role in spinal stenosis. Maintaining good posture helps to reduce the amount of strain on the spine, easing pressure on the spinal cord and spinal nerves.

Poor posture, on the other hand, can exacerbate spinal stenosis symptoms by increasing the amount of pressure on the spine. As a result, people with spinal stenosis need to maintain good posture, both when seated and when standing.

There are several ways to do this, including practicing proper alignment when sitting and standing, using supportive devices such as lumbar rolls, and avoiding high-impact activities that can jar the spine.

Use assistive devices: Spinal stenosis can be aggravated by activities such as walking or standing for long periods. However, using a cane or walker can help to relieve pressure on the spinal cord and reduce your risk of falling. In addition, using a cane or walker can help you stay balanced and prevent you from over-exerting yourself. As a result, using a cane or walker can be an important part of managing your spinal stenosis.

LIFESTYLE REMEDIES TO MANAGE SPINAL STENOSIS

While there is no cure for spinal stenosis, there are some lifestyle remedies that can help to manage the symptoms. By following these tips, you can help to reduce the pain and discomfort associated with spinal stenosis and improve your quality of life.

Exercise: Exercise strengthens the muscles that support your spine, helping to prevent further compression of the nerves. Physical activity also helps to improve flexibility and range of motion, which can be limited in people with spinal stenosis. Regular exercise is one of the most important things you can do to manage your condition.

Walking: Walking is a low-impact form of exercise that can help to strengthen the muscles around your spine and improve your symptoms.

Stretching: Stretching helps to improve flexibility and range of motion. It is important to stretch before and after exercise to reduce your risk of injury.

Yoga: Yoga is a type of exercise that can help to improve flexibility, muscle strength, and balance. It is important to find a class that is specifically designed for people with spinal stenosis.

Swimming: Swimming is a great form of exercise for people with spinal stenosis because it helps to strengthen the muscles around your spine without putting any additional stress on the joints.

Eating a healthy diet: Eating a healthy diet is important for people with any chronic condition. A healthy diet can help to improve your overall health and reduce inflammation caused by spinal stenosis. Inflammation is a common symptom of spinal stenosis, and it can be aggravated by certain foods. Eating a diet that is high in anti-inflammatory foods can help to reduce inflammation and improve your overall health.

MANAGE SYMPTOMS OF SPINAL STENOSIS THROUGH DIET

There is no specific diet for people with spinal stenosis. However, eating a healthy diet can help you maintain a healthy weight and reduce inflammation. Additionally, avoiding foods that can trigger inflammation, such as processed foods, sugar, and refined carbs, can help to minimize symptoms.

Foods to Eat

Anti-inflammatory foods: Anti-inflammatory foods are becoming more popular as people become more aware of the link between inflammation and disease. Spinal stenosis, for example, is a condition that is caused by inflammation of the spinal cord. By eating anti-inflammatory foods, you can help to reduce the inflammation that is causing your condition.

Some of the best anti-inflammatory foods include omega-3 fatty acids, turmeric, ginger, and green leafy vegetables. All of these foods contain compounds that have been shown to reduce inflammation in the body.

In addition, they are all incredibly healthy foods that can provide other benefits, such as improving heart health or boosting cognitive function. So, if you are looking to reduce inflammation in your body, be sure to add these anti-inflammatory foods to your diet.

Fruits and vegetables: These nutrient-rich foods contain antioxidants that can help reduce inflammation. They also provide fiber, which can help reduce constipation and promote regularity. In addition, fruits and vegetables are low in calories and fat, making them a good choice for people who are trying to lose weight. Including more of these healthy foods in your diet may help to ease your spinal stenosis symptoms.

Healthy fats: A healthy diet that includes healthy fats can help to reduce inflammation and pain associated with spinal stenosis. Healthy fats are found in olive oil, avocados, nuts, and seeds. Including these foods in your diet can help to improve your overall health and well-being.

Foods to Avoid

Processed foods: Processed foods are high in sugar and unhealthy fats, which can trigger inflammation. Inflammation is a natural response of the body to injury or infection, but chronic inflammation can lead to various health problems. Spinal stenosis is often caused by chronic inflammation, which can damage the spine over time. Therefore, eating a diet full of processed foods can increase your risk of developing this condition.

Sugar: Sugar can also cause inflammation and contribute to weight gain. Sugar enters the bloodstream and triggers an inflammatory response from the body. This response can cause swelling, pain, and stiffness.

In addition, sugar can interfere with the body's ability to absorb nutrients, leading to weight gain. While sugar is not the only cause of these conditions, it can play a role in their development. Therefore, it is important to be aware of the potential risks of consuming too much sugar.

Refined carbs: Refined carbs are found in foods like white bread, pasta, and rice. These foods have been stripped of their outer bran and germ, leaving only the starchy endosperm. This process not only removes important vitamins and minerals but also increases the glycemic index of these foods, causing spikes in blood sugar levels. Over time, high blood sugar levels can damage the spinal cord, leading to spinal stenosis.

Including these nutrients in your diet through food or supplements can help to improve your symptoms.

SAMPLE RECIPES

Vegan Caribbean Bowl

Ingredients:

- 1 cup jasmine rice
- 1 cup coconut milk
- 1 cup broth
- 1 tsp. salt
- 1/4 cup unsweetened dried coconut flakes, shredded
- 4 leaves kale or collard greens, stems removed and sliced thinly
- 1/4 white cabbage, shredded
- 1/2 red bell pepper, julienned
- 1 lime, halved
- 1 tbsp. coconut oil
- 1/2 orange
- Optional: 1-2 tsp. sesame oil
- Optional, choices for garnish: avocado, carrot, cilantro lime, orange, pineapple, and/or scallion, may be combined or not

Marinade:

- 1/2 cup fresh squeezed orange juice
- 1/4 cup soy sauce
- 1 tbsp. jerk seasoning
- 1 tsp. toasted sesame oil (Asian variety)
- tempeh, cubed or sliced (may also use other protein sources if desired)

Instructions:

For the marinade:

1. Mix all the marinade ingredients.
2. Throw in the tempeh in the marinade. Let it soak for at least half an hour.
3. In a saucepan, pour in the rice, coconut milk, broth, coconut flakes, and salt.
4. Set to medium-high heat and leave to boil.
5. Lower heat and allow to simmer for about 20 minutes, covered.
6. Once done, turn off the heat and leave the rice for now.
7. In a bowl, put red pepper, kale, and cabbage. Squeeze half a lime over.
8. In a pan placed over medium-high heat, pour in coconut oil.
9. Add the marinated tempeh to the hot oil. Cook until all sides are cooked well.
10. Add a teaspoon or two of sesame oil if desired. Squeeze in half an orange.
11. Remove tempeh from the pan.
12. In a serving bowl, scoop in rice, tempeh, and vegetables.

13. Upon serving, garnish according to your preference.

Baked Flounder

Ingredients:

- 1 lb. flounder, filleted
- 1/4 tsp. salt
- 1 cup halved red grapes
- 1 tbsp. extra-virgin olive oil
- 2 tbsp. parsley, chopped finely
- 1 tbsp. lemon juice
- 1 cup almonds, chopped and toasted
- freshly ground black pepper, to taste

Instructions:

1. Preheat the oven to 375°F.
2. Place fish on a sheet tray. Season with olive oil, salt, and pepper.
3. Combine the almonds, grapes, lemon juice, parsley, 1-1/2 tsp. of olive oil, 1/8 tsp of salt, and black pepper in a bowl.
4. Bake the fish for about 3 minutes.
5. Flip the fish and return to the oven.
6. Bake for another 3 minutes, or until the fish is starting to flake, while the center is still translucent. Don't overcook.
7. Serve immediately, topped with the grape mixture.

Salmon with Avocados and Brussels Sprouts

Ingredients:

- 2 lbs. of salmon filet, divided into 4 pieces
- 1 tsp. ground cumin
- 1 tsp. onion powder
- 1 tsp. paprika powder
- 1/2 tsp. garlic powder
- 1 tsp. chili powder
- Himalayan sea salt
- black pepper, freshly ground

Avocado sauce:

- 2 chopped avocados
- 1 lime, squeezed for the juice
- 1 tbsp. extra-virgin olive oil
- 1 tbsp. fresh minced cilantro
- 1 diced small red onion
- 1 minced garlic clove
- Himalayan sea salt to taste
- black pepper, freshly ground

Brussels sprout:

- 3 lbs. of Brussels Sprout
- 1/2 cup raw honey
- 1/2 cup balsamic vinegar

- 1/2 cup melted coconut oil
- 1 cup dried cranberries
- Himalayan sea salt
- black pepper, freshly ground

Instructions:

To make the salmon and avocado sauce:

1. Combine cumin, onion, chili powder, garlic, and paprika seasoned with salt and pepper. Mix well before dry rubbing on the salmon.
2. Place the salmon in the fridge for 30 minutes.
3. Preheat the grill.
4. In a bowl, mash avocado until the texture becomes smooth. Pour in all the remaining ingredients and mix thoroughly.
5. Grill salmon for 5 minutes on each side or until cooked.
6. Drizzle avocado on cooked salmon.

To prepare the Brussels Sprouts:

1. Preheat the oven to 375°F.
2. Mix Brussels Sprouts with coconut oil. Season with salt and pepper.
3. Place vegetables on a baking sheet and roast for about 30 minutes.
4. In a separate pan, combine vinegar and honey.
5. Simmer in slow heat until it boils and thickens.
6. Drizzle them on top of the Brussels Sprouts.
7. Serve with the salmon.

Kale Fried Rice

Ingredients:

- 2 tbsp. coconut oil
- 2 whole eggs
- 2 large garlic cloves, minced
- 3 large green onions, thinly sliced
- 1 cup of carrots, cut into matchsticks
- 1 cup of Brussels sprouts, diced
- 1 medium bunch of kale, ribs removed and the leaves shredded
- 2 cups brown rice, cooked and cooled
- 1/4 tsp. Himalayan salt
- 1/4 cup of lemon balm leaves, diced
- 3/4 cups of shredded coconut, unsweetened variety
- fresh cilantro, for garnishing

Instructions:

1. Heat a teaspoon of oil in a large skillet over medium-high heat.
2. Pour in the egg mixture.
3. Cook the eggs while occasionally stirring.
4. Remove from the pan and set aside.
5. Pour another teaspoon of coconut oil into the pan, along with Brussels sprouts, carrots, garlic, and green onions.
6. Stir now and then until the vegetables look tender.
7. Add kale and salt.
8. Remove from the pan and put them into where the egg is.

9. Put the remaining coconut oil into the pan. Add in
   coconut flakes, stirring frequently
10. Add rice and stir it in.
11. Add the egg and vegetable mixture to the pan, as well as
   the lemon balm leaves.
12. Stir to combine and heat through.
13. Transfer to a serving bowl and garnish with fresh
   cilantro.
14. Serve and enjoy.

Asian-Themed Macrobiotic Bowl

Ingredients:

- 2 cups cooked quinoa
- 4 carrots
- 1 package of smoked tofu
- 1 tbsp. nutritional yeast
- 2 tbsp. coconut aminos
- 4 tbsp. sunflower sprouts
- 2 tbsp. fermented vegetables
- 1 cup of shiitake mushrooms
- 1 avocado
- 2 tbsp. hemp seeds
- 2-3 cooked beets
- coconut oil cooking spray

Dressing:

- 2 tbsp. miso paste

- 1 tbsp. tahini
- 1 clove of garlic, crushed
- 1 tbsp. olive oil
- 1/2 lime, juiced
- 3 tbsp. water

Instructions:

1. Roast the carrots in the oven at 400°F for 30-40 minutes.
2. Wash the vegetables, trim, and spray them with coconut oil.
3. Add them to the oven. When they are cooked, set them aside till you are ready to assemble the Buddha bowl.
4. Make the dressing by combining all of the ingredients in a medium-sized bowl. If the dressing appears lumpy, add more water.
5. To build the bowl, put the quinoa on the bottom and then arrange the vegetables on top.
6. Sprinkle the bowls with hemp seeds and drizzle the dressing over top.
7. Now serve and enjoy!

Chicken Salad

Ingredients:

- 1 small can of premium chunk chicken breast packed in water
- 1 stalk celery, large, finely chopped
- 1/4 cup reduced-fat mayonnaise

- 4 romaine leaves or red leaf lettuce, washed and trimmed
- 2 oz. blue cheese, crumbled
- 8 pcs. cherry tomatoes or 1 ripe tomato, quartered
- 1 cucumber, small and sliced thinly

Instructions:

1. Drain canned chicken and transfer to a bowl.
2. Put in celery and mayonnaise.
3. Mix lightly. Don't crush the chicken.
4. In a separate shallow bowl, place the lettuce neatly.
5. Add the chicken salad in the middle and sprinkle blue cheese over it.
6. Add tomatoes and cucumber slices to the plate.
7. Refrigerate before serving, cover with plastic wrap.

Baked Salmon

Ingredients:

- 2 salmon fillets
- 6 cups of fresh spinach
- 2 tsp. coconut oil
- 1/4 tsp. garlic powder
- 1/4 tsp. turmeric
- 3 large cloves of garlic
- lemon juice
- salt
- pepper

Instructions:

1. Preheat the oven to 400°F.
2. Line a baking dish with parchment paper.
3. Marinate salmon fillets in lemon juice, coconut oil, garlic powder, turmeric, salt, and pepper.
4. Let it sit for a few minutes. This may also be done the night before to help the juices and flavor get into the salmon.
5. Once the oven is ready, bake the salmon for 15 minutes.
6. Cook some of the garlic in a pan with coconut oil.
7. Add spinach and cook until ready. Season with salt and pepper to taste.
8. Take salmon out of the oven and put spinach beside it.
9. Serve and enjoy.

Asian Zucchini Salad

Ingredients:

- 1 medium zucchini, sliced thinly into spirals
- 1/3 cup rice vinegar
- 3/4 cup avocado oil
- 1 cup sunflower seeds, shells removed
- 1 lb. cabbage, shredded
- 1 tsp. stevia drops
- 1 cup of almonds, sliced

Instructions:

1. Cut the zucchini spirals into smaller parts. Set aside.

2. Put almonds, sunflower seeds, and cabbage in a large bowl. Combine the ingredients well.
3. Add zucchini to the mixture.
4. In a small bowl, mix vinegar, stevia, and oil using a whisk or fork.
5. Pour the vinegar mixture all over the zucchini mixture. Toss well. Make sure everything is covered with the dressing.
6. Refrigerate for 2 hours before serving.

Low FODMAP Burger

Ingredients:

- 1-1/4 lbs. ground pork
- 1/4 tsp. allspice
- 1/2 tsp. salt
- 1/2 tsp. white pepper
- 1/2 tsp. ground nutmeg
- 1/2 tsp. caraway seeds
- 1/2 tsp. ground ginger

Instructions:

1. Preheat the grill then prepare the patty.
2. Using a small mixing bowl, stir together the salt, pepper, allspice, nutmeg, and ginger until fully combined.
3. Place the ground in a large mixing bowl and add the spice mixture.

4. Mix thoroughly until spices are evenly distributed to the pork.
5. Make round, flat burger patties using the palm of your hands.
6. Grill the patties and serve with gluten-free buns and mustard sauce.

Stir-Fried Cabbage and Apples

Ingredients:

- 1 shallot, thinly sliced
- 1/2 apple, cut into cubes
- 1/4 savoy cabbage, sliced thinly into strips
- 3–4 radishes, sliced thinly
- 1/2–1 tsp. coconut oil
- salt, to taste

Instructions:

1. Pour some coconut oil into a wok.
2. Add shallot and cook until translucent.
3. Add the cabbage, radish, and apples to the wok.
4. Stir-fry for about 5 minutes. Don't overcook.
5. Add salt to taste.
6. Serve while warm.

Asparagus and Greens Salad with Tahini and Poppy Seed Dressing

Ingredients:

- 10 to 12 asparagus stalks, washed well and sliced into ribbons
- 5 radishes, washed well, and sliced thinly
- 2 to 3 rainbow carrots, peeled and sliced thinly
- 1 handful of wild spinach
- 1 small handful of microgreens, washed well
- 1 small handful of sunflower greens, washed well
- optional: a few pieces of chive blossoms

For the dressing:

- 2 tbsp. tahini
- 1 tbsp. poppy seeds
- 1 tbsp. extra-virgin olive oil
- salt
- pepper

Instructions:

1. For the dressing, whisk ingredients together in a small bowl.
2. In a separate bowl, toss salad ingredients into the mixture.
3. Drizzle dressing on salad upon serving.

Stir-Fried Cabbage and Apples

Ingredients:

- 1 shallot, thinly sliced

- 1/2 apple, cut into cubes
- 1/4 savoy cabbage, sliced thinly into strips
- 3–4 radishes, sliced thinly
- 1/2–1 tsp. coconut oil
- salt, to taste

Instructions:

1. Pour some coconut oil into a wok.
2. Add shallot and cook until translucent.
3. Add the cabbage, radish, and apples to the wok.
4. Stir-fry for about 5 minutes. Don't overcook.
5. Add salt to taste.
6. Serve while warm.

SUMMARY

Spinal stenosis is a condition that causes the narrowing of the spinal canal. This can lead to pain, numbness, and weakness in the legs and arms. In severe cases, paralysis can occur.

Spinal stenosis is typically diagnosed with imaging tests, such as an MRI or CT scan. Treatment depends on the severity of the condition and may include medications, physical therapy, epidural injections, or surgery.

There is no sure way to prevent spinal stenosis. However, maintaining a healthy weight, exercising regularly, and stopping smoking can help reduce your risk. There are also a few things you can do at home to help manage your symptoms, such as applying heat or ice, stretching, and practicing good posture. Eating a healthy diet can also help reduce inflammation.

If you think you may have spinal stenosis, it's important to see a doctor so they can diagnose and treat the condition. With proper treatment, many people with spinal stenosis can manage their symptoms and live a normal life.

FAQ About Spinal Stenosis

1. What are the two types of spinal stenosis?

There are two main types of spinal stenosis, the lumbar spine, and the cervical spine.

2. What are the symptoms of spinal stenosis?

The most common symptom of spinal stenosis is pain, which can range from mild to severe. Other symptoms include numbness, weakness, and tingling in the legs and arms. In severe cases, paralysis can occur.

3. What are the symptoms of severe spinal stenosis?

Severe spinal stenosis can cause paralysis. Other symptoms include severe pain, numbness, and weakness in the legs and arms.

4. How is spinal stenosis diagnosed?

Spinal stenosis is typically diagnosed with X-ray or imaging tests, such as an MRI or CT scan.

5. What are the treatment options for spinal stenosis?

Treatment depends on the severity of the condition and may include medications, physical therapy, epidural injections, or surgery.

6. How can I prevent spinal stenosis?

There is no sure way to prevent spinal stenosis. However, maintaining a healthy weight, exercising regularly, and stopping smoking can help reduce your risk. There are also a few things you can do at home to help manage your symptoms, such as applying heat or ice, stretching, and practicing good posture. Eating a healthy diet can also help reduce inflammation.

If you think you may have spinal stenosis, it's important to see a doctor so they can diagnose and treat the condition. With proper treatment, many people with spinal stenosis can manage their symptoms and live a normal life.

References

7 Foods You Need to Be Eating for Spinal Health | Comprehensive Spine. (n.d.). Comprehensive Spine Institute. Retrieved October 9, 2022, from https://www.csiortho.com/blog/2018/september/7-foods-you-need-to-be-eating-for-spinal-health/.

8 Foods for Spinal Health. (n.d.). Retrieved October 9, 2022, from https://www.spineuniverse.com/conditions/back-pain/8-foods-spinal-health.

Avoid These Foods During Back Pain. (2017, June 15). Texas Spine Clinic. https://www.texasspineclinic.com/foods-to-avoid-while-experiencing-back-pain/.

Guide | Physical Therapy Guide to Spinal Stenosis. (2018, January 8). Choose PT. https://www.choosept.com/guide/physical-therapy-guide-spinal-stenosis.

Lumbar Puncture (Spinal Tap)—Mayo Clinic. (n.d.). Retrieved October 9, 2022, from https://www.mayoclinic.org/tests-procedures/lumbar-puncture/about/pac-20394631.

Lumbar Spinal Stenosis—Orthoinfo—Aaos. (n.d.). Retrieved October 9, 2022, from https://www.orthoinfo.org/en/diseases--conditions/lumbar-spinal-stenosis/.

MD, G. C. (n.d.). Posture and Nutrition Adjustments for Lumbar Stenosis. Spine-Health. Retrieved October 9, 2022, from https://www.spine-health.com/conditions/spinal-stenosis/posture-and-nutrition-adjustments-lumbar-stenosis.

Spinal Stenosis. (n.d.). Retrieved October 9, 2022, from https://www.rheumatology.org/I-Am-A/Patient-Caregiver/Diseases-Conditions/Spinal-Stenosis.